COMPLETE GUIDE TO UNDERSTANDING COLONOSCOPY

Essential Tips, Preparation, Procedure Insights, Recovery, Post-Care For Optimal Digestive Health And Benefits Explained

KLEIN HOYLE

© [KLEIN HOYLE] [2024]

All rights reserved.

No part of this book may be reproduced, distributed, or transmitted in any form or by any means, including photocopying, recording, or other electronic or mechanical methods, without the publisher's prior written permission, with the exception of brief quotations in critical reviews and certain other noncommercial uses permitted by copyright law.

Disclaimer

The content in this book is based on the author's expertise and comprehension of the topic. The author has no affiliation or link with any corporation, business, or person. This book is meant to give general information and educational material only, and it should not be interpreted as professional medical advice. Always seek the advice of a skilled healthcare expert if you have any queries about medical issues or treatments. The author and publisher expressly disclaim any responsibility resulting directly or indirectly from the use or use of the information included in this book.

Table of Contents

CHAPTER 1 13
Introduction To Colonoscopy 13
What Is A Colonoscopy? 13
Why Are Colonoscopies Performed? 13
1. Screening: 13
2. Diagnostic: 14
Importance Of Early Detection And Prevention . 14
Common Misconceptions About Colonoscopies . 15
1. Uncomfortable Procedure: 15
2. Embarrassing or Invasive: 16
3. Unnecessary Procedure: 16

CHAPTER 2 19
Preparing For A Colonoscopy 19
Dietary Restriction And Bowel Preparation 19
Medication Adjustments Before The Procedure .. 20
Hygiene And Preparation Instructions 21
What To Expect During The Preparation Phase . 22

CHAPTER 3 25
Understanding The Procedure 25
Overview Of The Colonoscopy Procedure 25

Equipment For Colonoscopy 27
The Role Of Sedation In The Procedure 28
Potential Risks And Complications 30
   1. Bleeding: 30
   2. Perforation: 30
   3. Sedation-related adverse reactions: 30
   4. Incomplete examination: 31
   5. Infection: 31

CHAPTER 4 33
The Day Of Colonoscopy 33
The Arrival And Registration Process 33
Pre-Procedure Consultation With Medical Staff. 34
Administration Of Sedation And Anesthesia 36
Pre-Procedure Check And Preparation 37

CHAPTER 5 39
During Colonoscopy 39
Positioning For The Procedure 39
Insertion Of The Colonoscope 40
Visualization Of The Colon 40
Biopsy And Polyp Removal Process 41

CHAPTER 6 43

Post-Colonoscopy Care 43
Recovery Process At The Facility 43
Potential Side Effects And How To Manage Them
.... 44
    1. Bloating and Gas: 44
    3. Rectal Bleeding: 45
    4. Sedation response: 45
Diet And Activity Recommendations Following
The Procedure 46
    1. Hydration: 46
    2. Light food: 46
    3. Gradual Return to Normal Diet: 46
Follow-Up Instructions And Appointments 47
    1. Results Discussion: 47
    2. Medication adjustments: 48
    3. Future Screenings: 48
    4. Addressing issues or Questions: 48
CHAPTER 7 51
Understanding Colonoscopy Results 51
Interpreting Results From The Operation 51

- Different Categories Of Results: Normal, Abnormal, And Inconclusive 52
- An Explanation Of Popular Words And Diagnoses 53
- What To Do Next Based On The Results? 54

CHAPTER 8 57
- The Benefits And Importance Of Colonoscopy ..57
- Colonoscopy's Role In Preventing Colorectal Cancer 57
- Early Detection Of Polyps And Other Abnormalities 59
- Comparison Of Other Screening Methods 60
- Long-Term Health Benefits And Implications ...62

CHAPTER 9 65
- Special Considerations And FAQ 65
- Colonoscopy For Those With Certain Medical Issues 65
- Age Guidelines And Screening Frequency 67
- Addressing Frequent Worries And Anxieties 69
- Clearing Any Misunderstandings Regarding The Technique 72

CHAPTER 10 75

Moving Forward: Taking Control Of Your Health 75
The Need For Regular Screenings And Preventive Care 75
How To Maintain A Healthy Colon And Digestive System 77
Advocacy For Colon Cancer Awareness And Prevention 79
Resources For More Information And Support .. 81
Conclusion 83
THE END 87

ABOUT THIS BOOK

The "Complete Guide to Understanding Colonoscopy" is a wonderful resource for anybody looking to learn all there is to know about this important medical treatment. Beginning with an enlightening introduction, readers are introduced to the essential components of colonoscopies, including their purpose, importance in early detection, and refuting prevalent misunderstandings about them.

Chapter 2 dives into the critical preliminary measures needed in a colonoscopy. From dietary changes to precise cleanliness habits, this section methodically details the required preparations for a successful surgery. It also gives advice on medication modifications and a full summary of what to anticipate throughout the preparation period, all of which should alleviate any concerns readers may have.

Understanding the technique itself is critical, as Chapter 3 expertly demonstrates. It explains the details of a colonoscopy, from the equipment used to the function of sedation in improving patient comfort. Furthermore, possible risks and problems are extensively addressed, providing consumers with the information they need to make educated health choices.

On the day of the colonoscopy, Chapter 4 painstakingly walks readers through the whole procedure, from arrival and registration to pre-procedure consultations and sedation. This part attempts to reduce fear and build a feeling of preparation in patients by demystifying the procedure path.

During the colonoscopy, Chapter 5 explains the procedural details, such as patient positioning, colonoscope insertion, and visualization modalities. Furthermore, it throws light on the biopsy and polyp removal procedures, ensuring that readers understand each stage and its importance in diagnosing and avoiding colorectal disorders.

Post-colonoscopy care is also critical, as discussed in Chapter 6. This section provides extensive recommendations to ensure a comfortable post-procedural experience, including everything from the healing process to probable side effects and their treatment. It also makes food and exercise suggestions, stressing the need to follow through on follow-up instructions and visits for the best health results.

Understanding colonoscopy results is critical, and Chapter 7 provides readers with the information they need to appropriately interpret the findings. Individuals are empowered to take proactive steps based on their findings by clarifying various result kinds and explaining common words and diagnoses. This improves their general health and well-being.

Chapter 8 emphasizes the value and usefulness of colonoscopy in avoiding colorectal cancer and finding anomalies early. This section underlines the importance of colonoscopies in maintaining optimum health by comparing them to other screening procedures and emphasizing their long-term health effects.

Chapter 9 discusses special considerations and commonly asked issues for people with certain medical problems, as well as typical worries and misunderstandings. This section seeks to remove fears and increase trust in the process by offering clarity and reassurance.

Finally, Chapter 10 encourages readers to take responsibility for their health by promoting frequent screenings, living a healthy lifestyle, and spreading awareness about colon cancer prevention.

CHAPTER 1

Introduction To Colonoscopy

What Is A Colonoscopy?

A colonoscopy is a medical treatment that examines the inner lining of the large intestine (colon and rectal). It entails passing a flexible tube called a colonoscope through the anus and into the colon. The colonoscope features a small camera and light at the tip, which allows the clinician to observe the colon lining on a monitor.

Why Are Colonoscopies Performed?

Colonoscopies are typically used for two purposes: screening and diagnosis.

1. **Screening:** Individuals at medium risk of colorectal cancer should have frequent colonoscopies beginning at age 50, or earlier if they have a family history of

colorectal cancer or other risk factors. Screening detects colorectal cancer early when it is more curable, and it may also prevent cancer by eliminating precancerous polyps while the treatment is being performed.

2. Diagnostic: A colonoscopy may be conducted if a person exhibits symptoms such as rectal bleeding, changes in bowel habits, abdominal discomfort, or unexplained weight loss. In such circumstances, the technique assists the doctor in diagnosing problems such as colon cancer, inflammatory bowel disease (IBD), diverticulosis, or polyps.

Importance Of Early Detection And Prevention

Early diagnosis of colorectal cancer with screening colonoscopies may greatly enhance treatment results and survival rates. Colonoscopy, by finding and eliminating precancerous polyps during the operation, may prevent colorectal cancer from growing at all. This makes it an important weapon in the battle against colorectal cancer, one of the most frequent and lethal malignancies globally.

Colorectal cancer often develops without symptoms in its early stages, hence regular screening colonoscopies are suggested to detect it before symptoms occur. Precancerous polyps may be detected and removed before they develop into cancer, possibly saving lives.

Common Misconceptions About Colonoscopies

Despite its significance, various misunderstandings about colonoscopies may dissuade people from having them:

1. **Uncomfortable Procedure:** Many individuals are concerned that a colonoscopy may be uncomfortable. However, most patients are sedated to make them comfortable throughout the treatment, and they

usually experience no discomfort. Some may feel moderate soreness or cramps, although this is typically tolerable.

2. Embarrassing or Invasive: Some people are embarrassed or uncomfortable with the concept of having a tube placed into their rectum. Colonoscopy, on the other hand, is a common medical treatment that is conducted in secret and concerning qualified specialists. The advantages of early diagnosis and prevention significantly exceed any little inconvenience or embarrassment.

3. Unnecessary Procedure: Some people may assume that they do not need a colonoscopy if they do not have any symptoms or a family history of colorectal cancer. However, colorectal cancer may grow without symptoms, and many people who are diagnosed with it have no family history. Screening colonoscopies is advised for those at average risk to identify and prevent colorectal cancer early.

Addressing these misunderstandings and raising awareness about the value of colonoscopies will motivate more individuals to be screened and possibly save lives by diagnosing and preventing colorectal cancer.

CHAPTER 2

Preparing For A Colonoscopy

Dietary Restriction And Bowel Preparation

To achieve the best possible results from a colonoscopy, patients must follow stringent food restrictions and undergo bowel preparation. Before the colonoscopy, your doctor will give you specific instructions on what meals to avoid and how to prepare your intestine.

Typically, you will need to have a clear liquid diet for a day or two before the treatment. This might include drinking broth, clear liquids, gelatin, and simple tea or coffee without milk. It is important to avoid solid meals since they might leave residue in the colon, impeding the inspection procedure.

To fully cleanse your colon, you will also need to consume a bowel preparation solution. This solution, which is often a mix of polyethylene glycol and electrolytes, works by inducing diarrhea, and successfully emptying the colon of all feces and debris. While the flavor of the bowel preparation fluid may be unpleasant, it is critical that you drink it exactly as directed to have a successful colonoscopy.

Following the food restrictions and bowel preparation protocols religiously is critical for obtaining reliable findings during the colonoscopy. Failure to follow these guidelines may result in an incomplete examination or the need for a repeat operation, which may be inconvenient and pose health hazards.

Medication Adjustments Before The Procedure

In addition to food restrictions, you may need to modify your medication regimen before having a colonoscopy.

Certain medicines, such as blood thinners or anti-inflammatory drugs, might raise the possibility of bleeding during the surgery.

Your doctor will advise you on which drugs to continue taking and which to temporarily discontinue before the colonoscopy. you avoid difficulties, be sure you carefully follow these directions.

If you have any underlying health concerns or use drugs daily, you should consult with your doctor well before the treatment. They may provide tailored suggestions and change your medication schedule to guarantee your safety throughout the colonoscopy.

Hygiene And Preparation Instructions

Maintaining appropriate cleanliness and following preparation instructions are critical procedures before a colonoscopy. Your doctor will provide you with full advice on how to prepare for the surgery, including cleanliness habits and any special recommendations customized to your requirements.

You may be encouraged to wash or bathe the night before or the morning of your colonoscopy using a light soap. This ensures that your skin is clean and free of any impurities that may interfere with the treatment.

In addition to hygienic precautions, you must follow special preparation recommendations, such as avoiding certain skincare products, fragrances, or lotions that may interfere with the treatment. Adherence to these principles is critical to ensuring ideal circumstances for the colonoscopy and reducing the risk of complications.

What To Expect During The Preparation Phase

During the colonoscopy preparation phase, you should anticipate spending time adhering to food restrictions, drinking bowel preparation solutions, and emotionally and physically preparing for the operation.

It is common to feel hungry or exhausted while on a clear liquid diet and undergoing bowel preparation. To get the greatest results, remain hydrated and follow your doctor's directions.

You may have frequent bowel motions and diarrhea as a consequence of the bowel preparation solution. This is a typical aspect of the procedure that helps to properly clean the colon in preparation for the colonoscopy.

Overall, the colonoscopy preparatory step is critical to ensure the procedure's success. Following food restrictions, making medication changes as required, maintaining good cleanliness, and psychologically preparing oneself may all assist in guaranteeing a smooth and productive colonoscopy experience.

CHAPTER 3

Understanding The Procedure

Overview Of The Colonoscopy Procedure

A colonoscopy is a necessary procedure in which healthcare experts inspect the interior of your colon (large intestine) and rectum. Colorectal cancer screening is normally suggested for those over 50, although it may also be used to identify inflammatory bowel disease, polyps, and other gastrointestinal disorders. During the process, a colonoscope, or flexible tube with a camera attached, is introduced into the rectum and directed into the colon. This enables the doctor to visually examine the lining of your colon for any abnormalities.

The colonoscopy operation typically takes 30 to 60 minutes to perform, however, this might vary based on individual conditions.

Before the surgery, you will be given precise preparatory instructions to ensure that your colon is clear and free of blockages. This often entails following a watery diet and using laxatives to clear your intestines. When you arrive at the healthcare center, you will be given sedation to help you relax and avoid pain throughout the treatment.

During the colonoscopy, you'll lay on your side while the doctor carefully inserts and advances the colonoscope. The camera at the tip of the colonoscope feeds pictures to a display, enabling the doctor to thoroughly inspect the lining of your colon. If any abnormalities are discovered, such as polyps or inflammation, the doctor may obtain tissue samples (biopsies) for further examination. In certain circumstances, polyps may be removed during the surgery to lower the risk of colorectal cancer.

When the examination is done, the colonoscope is gradually removed, and the operation is completed. You may suffer bloating or gas afterward, although this normally goes away fast. The doctor will share their results with you and make any suggestions for further treatment or follow-up.

Equipment For Colonoscopy

The colonoscopy is the principal tool used during a colonoscopy. This is a long, flexible tube with a small camera and light source at its tip. The colonoscope also has passages for conveying air and water, as well as extra tools for biopsy or polyp removal if required. The colonoscope's flexibility enables it to easily negotiate the twists and turns of the colon.

In addition to the colonoscope, additional equipment utilized during a colonoscopy includes a monitor to show the pictures collected by the camera, as well as different attachments such as air pumps and suction devices to help with the inspection. These technologies serve to enable good visibility of the colon and permit any necessary procedures.

Modern colonoscopes use high-definition cameras and sophisticated imaging technology, allowing for a thorough study of the colon lining. Some colonoscopes have features like narrow-band imaging (NBI) and chromoendoscopy, which can identify subtle abnormalities such as tiny polyps or inflammation.

Overall, the equipment used during a colonoscopy is meticulously engineered to give excellent visibility and flexibility, enabling physicians to conduct complete inspections and procedures with accuracy and safety.

The Role Of Sedation In The Procedure

Sedation is an important part of the colonoscopy treatment since it keeps patients comfortable and calm during the test. Most colonoscopies are conducted under conscious sedation, often known as twilight sedation, which includes delivering medicines to produce relaxation and sleepiness while keeping the patient awake and alert.

Conscious sedation during a colonoscopy is often achieved with a mix of sedative and analgesic drugs. These drugs are often given intravenously by a qualified healthcare professional. The sedative reduces anxiety and promotes serenity, and the analgesic reduces discomfort or agony during the treatment.

Conscious sedation is favored for colonoscopies because it enables patients to participate in the procedure while reducing pain and anxiety. Unlike general anesthetic, conscious sedation has fewer dangers and adverse effects, allowing for a faster recovery period.

Throughout the treatment, the healthcare team will continuously monitor your vital signs to guarantee your safety and change the dose of sedation as necessary. After the colonoscopy, the sedative effects will gradually wear off, and you will be watched in a recovery room until you are completely awake and can handle fluids.

Potential Risks And Complications

While colonoscopy is usually regarded as a safe operation, it does contain certain risks and possible consequences, which are uncommon. This may include:

1. Bleeding: When a biopsy or polyp is removed during a colonoscopy, bleeding may occur. The majority of bleeding is minimal and resolves on its own, but in rare circumstances, further intervention may be necessary to control the bleeding.

2. Perforation: There is a slight possibility of the colon or rectum becoming perforated during colonoscopy. Perforation is a significant condition that may need surgery for correction.

3. Sedation-related adverse reactions: Some people may develop side effects or allergic responses to the sedative drugs. These may include nausea, vomiting, allergic responses, or respiratory depression.

However, such responses are uncommon and may be handled by a healthcare team.

4. Incomplete examination: In certain situations, the colonoscopy may be unable to be completed owing to technological issues or patient variables such as severe colon inflammation or narrowed colon segments. If this happens, more imaging tests or a repeat colonoscopy may be required.

5. Infection: While uncommon, there is a small risk of infection related to colonoscopy, especially if tissue samples or polyps are removed. The danger of infection is reduced by adhering to stringent sterile procedures and utilizing disposable equipment.

Before getting a colonoscopy, you should address any concerns or medical issues with your doctor to confirm that the operation is right for you. To ensure the colonoscopy's safety and efficacy, carefully follow all preparatory instructions.

CHAPTER 4

The Day Of Colonoscopy

The Arrival And Registration Process

On the day of your colonoscopy, you will usually arrive at the medical institution or hospital at a certain time. This arrival time is normally scheduled in advance to allow for essential preparations and to ensure the operation runs successfully. Arriving on time enables the medical personnel to stick to their schedule and saves you from needless waiting time.

Upon arrival, you will go through a registration procedure identical to that of a routine doctor's appointment or hospital admittance. This includes supplying your personal information, medical history, and insurance information, if applicable. The staff will walk you through the procedure and may ask you to complete any papers.

After completing the registration process, you will be escorted to a waiting room, where you may be required to change into a hospital gown or other suitable apparel. This is often done to ensure your comfort throughout the surgery and to provide the medical staff with easier access.

During this period, it is usual to experience a range of feelings, including worry and anxiety. Remember that the medical team are seasoned experts who conduct colonoscopies daily and will do their utmost to keep you comfortable and safe during the procedure.

Pre-Procedure Consultation With Medical Staff

Before the colonoscopy process starts, you will have the chance to chat with the medical personnel who will be caring for you. This might include the gastroenterologist doing the colonoscopy, nurses, anesthesiologists, and any other healthcare personnel who will be present throughout the operation.

During these sessions, you will be able to ask any questions you have regarding the process, voice any concerns, and go over any special instructions or preparations. It is critical to be open and honest throughout these conversations so that the medical team can give you the best possible treatment.

The medical professionals will also go over your medical history and any pre-existing illnesses you may have. This information allows them to personalize the treatment and anesthetic delivery to your specific requirements, assuring your safety and comfort throughout.

If you have any allergies or drug reactions, please let us know during these appointments. This enables the medical team to take essential safeguards and make changes to the operation plan as required.

Administration Of Sedation And Anesthesia

Sedation or anesthesia is an important part of a colonoscopy because it ensures your comfort throughout the operation. The kind and dose of sedation used will be determined by many criteria, including your medical history, age, and the intricacy of the treatment.

An anesthesiologist or nurse anesthetist will usually provide sedation intravenously. The medicine causes relaxation and sleepiness, helping you to be comfortable and motionless throughout the colonoscopy. In rare situations, you may be given a mix of sedatives and pain medicines to increase your comfort.

It is critical to follow any fasting recommendations given by your healthcare professional before the surgery, as this reduces the chance of issues related to anesthetic delivery.

The medical staff will continuously monitor you during the sedation procedure to guarantee your safety and well-being. They will monitor your vital indicators, such as heart rate, blood pressure, and oxygen levels, during the treatment.

Pre-Procedure Check And Preparation

Before the colonoscopy, the medical team will do several pre-procedure exams and preparations to verify that everything is in order. This may entail validating your identification, clarifying procedure information, and going over any last-minute instructions.

The gastroenterologist may also do a quick physical examination, concentrating on your abdomen and rectal region. This allows them to analyze your general health and detect any possible difficulties that may impact the treatment.

In certain circumstances, a mild enema may be used to empty the colon of any leftover feces or debris. This step is often performed immediately before the colonoscopy and improves the visibility of the intestinal lining during the examination.

Once all of the essential examinations and preparations have been completed, you will be brought to the procedure room for the colonoscopy. The medical staff will walk you through each stage of the procedure, ensuring your comfort and safety throughout.

CHAPTER 5

During Colonoscopy

Positioning For The Procedure

Before the colonoscopy, you will be requested to change into a hospital gown and take off any jewelry or accessories. You will next be positioned on your left side, legs brought up to your chest. This posture straightens out the colon, allowing the doctor to traverse the scope across the whole length of the large intestine.

Before beginning the treatment, the medical team will evaluate your vital signs and make sure you are comfortable. They will also offer sedation or anesthetic if necessary to help you relax and relieve pain.

Insertion Of The Colonoscope

With you in the appropriate posture, the doctor will gently slide the lubricated, flexible colonoscope into your rectum. The colonoscope is a long, thin tube with a light and camera connected to the tip, which allows the doctor to look within your colon in real-time.

As the colonoscope moves slowly through the colon, the doctor will carefully navigate it around bends and curves to ensure a complete inspection of the whole length of the large intestine. During the insertion procedure, the medical team will interact with you and check your comfort level, modifying sedation as needed.

Visualization Of The Colon

As the colonoscope moves, the camera at its tip delivers high-definition photos to a display, enabling the doctor to see the interior of your colon in great detail.

The scans let the doctor discover any abnormalities in the gut lining, such as inflammation, polyps, or tumors.

The doctor will also inflate the colon with air or carbon dioxide to extend the walls and provide a clearer view of the interior surface. This inflation may cause you to feel pressure or bloating, but it allows the doctor to better maneuver the scope and spot any abnormalities.

During the visualization process, the doctor may capture still photographs or video recordings of any worrisome locations to be analyzed or documented.

Biopsy And Polyp Removal Process

If the doctor finds any abnormal tissue, such as polyps or suspicious lesions, during the colonoscopy, they may do a biopsy or remove it right away.

A biopsy is the process of removing a tiny sample of tissue from an abnormal location using specialized instruments that are passed via the colonoscope. This tissue sample is then submitted to a laboratory for testing to determine if it is benign or malignant.

Similarly, polyps, or abnormal growths on the colon lining, may be removed during the colonoscopy process. The doctor will use small devices pushed through the colonoscope to remove the polyps, a procedure called polypectomy. Removing polyps not only enables for study under a microscope but also minimizes the likelihood that they may grow into cancer over time.

Following any biopsies or polyp removals, the doctor will thoroughly inspect the whole colon again to verify that no abnormalities are overlooked. After the surgery, the colonoscope is gently removed and you are escorted to a recovery room to relax while the anesthesia wears off.

CHAPTER 6

Post-Colonoscopy Care

Recovery Process At The Facility

Following your colonoscopy, you will be sent to a recovery room, where medical personnel will monitor you until you are completely awake and conscious. This procedure usually takes 30 minutes to an hour. The sedative used during the surgery may cause you to feel groggy or drowsy during this time. It is common to feel confused or tired, but these symptoms will eventually fade.

Your vital indicators, such as blood pressure, heart rate, and respiration, will be continuously checked to prevent problems. You may also be given fluids intravenously to help you rehydrate if required. The medical staff will evaluate your health and give any necessary treatment or drugs.

Once you're completely awake and stable, you'll be able to return home with a competent adult. Due to the lingering effects of sedation, it is not safe to drive or operate equipment for at least 24 hours following the treatment.

Potential Side Effects And How To Manage Them

While colonoscopy is a reasonably safe operation, you may suffer some side effects afterward. These may include:

1. Bloating and Gas: The air pushed into your colon during the inspection may cause you to feel bloated or gassy after the operation. This soreness should subside within a few hours when you pass gas.

2. Mild abdominal pain is usual after a colonoscopy. This is often transitory and may be treated with over-the-counter pain relievers such as ibuprofen or acetaminophen.

3. **Rectal Bleeding:** Minor rectal bleeding or spotting may occur, particularly if polyps were removed during the treatment. This is generally mild and should resolve on its own within a day or two. If the bleeding continues or is severe, call your doctor right away.

4. **Sedation response:** In rare situations, patients may have an adverse response to the sedative medicines used during the surgery. Symptoms may include nausea, vomiting, disorientation, and trouble breathing. If you have any severe or persistent symptoms, get medical treatment right once.

To alleviate these side effects, keep hydrated, relax, and avoid intense activity for the rest of the day. If you have any concerns, or if symptoms continue or worsen, please contact your healthcare professional for additional assistance.

Diet And Activity Recommendations Following The Procedure

Following your colonoscopy, your doctor will provide specific dietary and exercise suggestions to help you recuperate and avoid issues. This may include:

1. Hydration: Stay hydrated by drinking lots of fluids, such as water, clear soups, and electrolyte-rich drinks, which can help flush out any lingering gas or sedative medicines.

2. Light food: For the first day or two after the surgery, eat light, readily digested food. This might include items like broth-based soups, crackers, bread, yogurt, and cooked veggies. Avoid heavy or spicy meals that may irritate your digestive tract.

3. Gradual Return to Normal Diet: As you feel better, slowly reintroduce solid meals into your diet. To encourage good digestion, eat foods high in fiber such as fruits, vegetables, whole grains, and lean meats.

4. Avoidance of Certain Foods: Some foods may aggravate bloating or gas, so avoid them temporarily. Carbonated drinks, beans, cabbage, broccoli, and dairy products are all examples of lactose-intolerant foods.

5. Rest and avoid strenuous activities for the rest of the day after your colonoscopy. Avoid heavy lifting, intense exercise, and other activities that may strain your abdominal muscles.

Follow-Up Instructions And Appointments

Before you leave the facility, your doctor will give you follow-up instructions and arrange any required visits. This may include:

1. **Results Discussion:** Your doctor will go over the results of the colonoscopy with you, including any abnormalities, polyps, or other difficulties discovered during the operation.

They will explain how these results affect your health and any necessary follow-up treatment.

2. Medication adjustments: If polyps were removed during the colonoscopy or if any other abnormalities were discovered, your doctor may prescribe new drugs or propose adjustments to your existing ones to address any underlying conditions or avoid future difficulties.

3. Future Screenings: Based on your age, medical history, and colonoscopy findings, your doctor will propose a timetable for future colon cancer screenings. This might include frequent colonoscopies or other screening procedures to check your colon health and spot any changes early.

4. Addressing issues or Questions: If you have any issues or questions concerning the operation, healing process, or follow-up treatment, please contact your doctor or healthcare team for answers.

They're there to help you and make sure you have all the knowledge you need to take care of yourself properly.

Following these post-colonoscopy care guidelines and attending any follow-up consultations as directed will help maintain optimum healing, monitor colon health, and lower your risk of colorectal cancer and other gastrointestinal disorders.

CHAPTER 7

Understanding Colonoscopy Results

Interpreting Results From The Operation

Following a colonoscopy, it is critical to comprehend the findings to provide appropriate follow-up care and treatment. Your healthcare professional will present you with a report detailing the procedure's results. This report will normally contain information about the health of your colon, any anomalies discovered, and suggestions for further steps.

Understanding the visual inspection of the colon is critical for interpreting colonoscopy findings. During the process, the gastroenterologist carefully examines the colon's lining using a flexible tube connected to a camera. They check for indications of inflammation, polyps, ulcers, and other abnormalities. The results are recorded and discussed in the procedure report.

Different Categories Of Results: Normal, Abnormal, And Inconclusive

Colonoscopy findings may be divided into three categories: normal, abnormal, and inconclusive.

A normal result means that the gastroenterologist found no abnormalities in the colon. This is comforting and indicates that your colon is healthy, with no evidence of illness or precancerous growths.

An abnormal result indicates that the gastroenterologist found anything uncommon during the surgery. This might include the existence of polyps, which are growths on the colon's inner lining that, if not treated, can progress to cancer. Other anomalies may include inflammation, ulceration, or infection symptoms.

A colonoscopy may sometimes provide unclear results. This indicates that the gastroenterologist was unable to adequately view certain sections of the colon owing to reasons such as inadequate stool preparation or anatomical limitations. In such circumstances, further tests or procedures may be required to provide a more accurate evaluation of the colon.

An Explanation Of Popular Words And Diagnoses

Understanding the language used in colonoscopy reports is critical for interpreting the results. Here are some typical words and diagnoses you may come across:

• Polyps are tiny growths on the inner lining of the colon. While the majority of polyps are benign, if not removed, some may progress to malignancy.

• Inflammation in the colon may suggest inflammatory bowel disease (IBD), such as Crohn's or ulcerative colitis.

• Ulcers are sores or lesions on the lining of the colon. They may be caused by a variety of circumstances, such as infection or inflammation.

• Diverticula are tiny pouches that may occur in the colon. They are widespread, particularly as individuals age, and seldom produce symptoms until they become irritated or infected.

Your healthcare professional will clarify any terminology or diagnoses indicated in your colonoscopy report and discuss their implications for your health.

What To Do Next Based On The Results?

The proper next actions after a colonoscopy will be determined by the results of the operation.

• If the findings are normal, your healthcare professional may suggest a follow-up colonoscopy in a few years based on your age and risk factors.

- If polyps are found during a colonoscopy, your gastroenterologist may remove them or arrange a separate surgery.

- If inflammation or other indications indicate an underlying problem, more testing or therapy may be required to control and avoid consequences.

It is important to follow your healthcare provider's instructions for follow-up treatment and screening to preserve colon health and spot possible problems early. Regular colonoscopies are an important tool for avoiding colon cancer and maintaining good gastrointestinal health.

CHAPTER 8

The Benefits And Importance Of Colonoscopy

Colonoscopy's Role In Preventing Colorectal Cancer

Colorectal cancer is a major public health problem worldwide, but the good news is that it is largely preventable with early identification and treatment. Colonoscopy is important in avoiding colorectal cancer because it allows physicians to discover and remove precancerous growths known as polyps before they develop into cancerous tumors.

During a colonoscopy, a thin, flexible tube with a small camera is introduced into the rectum and advanced across the colon. This lets the doctor thoroughly inspect the colon's lining for any abnormalities, such as polyps or cancers.

If polyps are discovered, they may be removed during the surgery, lowering the risk of colorectal cancer.

Colonoscopy is useful in avoiding colorectal cancer because it detects and removes polyps early on. The majority of colorectal malignancies develop from precancerous polyps over time, offering a chance for intervention. Removing these polyps during a colonoscopy dramatically reduces the risk of cancer development.

Regular colonoscopy screening is suggested for those at average risk of colorectal cancer, which commonly begins around the age of 50. Those with a family history of colorectal cancer or certain genetic abnormalities, on the other hand, may need to start screening sooner and at a higher frequency.

Early Detection Of Polyps And Other Abnormalities

One of the basic purposes of colonoscopy is to identify polyps and other abnormalities in the colon. Polyps are growths that protrude from the colon's inner lining and may be of various sizes and shapes. While most polyps are innocuous, some have the potential to become cancerous over time.

During a colonoscopy, the doctor uses the endoscope's camera to thoroughly check the colon for polyps. If polyps are discovered, they may be removed using specialist devices inserted via the endoscope. The removal procedure, known as polypectomy, is typically fast and painless.

In addition to polyps, colonoscopy may identify other abnormalities in the colon, such as inflammation, ulcers, and malignancies. Early diagnosis of these anomalies enables timely treatment and management, lowering the risk of complications and improving patient outcomes.

Regular colonoscopy screening is critical for early diagnosis of polyps and other abnormalities, particularly in those at increased risk of colorectal cancer. Colonoscopy, by detecting these anomalies early on, may help prevent colorectal cancer and enhance overall health.

Comparison Of Other Screening Methods

Colorectal cancer may be detected using a variety of screening procedures, including stool tests, flexible sigmoidoscopy, and computed tomography (CT) colonography. While each approach has merits and disadvantages, colonoscopy is still the gold standard for colorectal cancer screening owing to its high sensitivity and ability to identify and remove polyps in the same session.

Stool-based diagnostics, such as fecal occult blood tests (FOBT) and fecal immunochemical tests (FIT), are non-invasive procedures for detecting blood in the stool, which may indicate colorectal cancer or polyps. However, these tests may miss certain polyps or malignancies, necessitating a subsequent colonoscopy for additional investigation.

Flexible sigmoidoscopy is another screening approach that includes introducing a flexible tube into the rectum to inspect the colon's lower portion. Flexible sigmoidoscopy may identify abnormalities in the lower colon, but it does not offer a comprehensive picture of the colon and may miss polyps or tumors in the upper colon.

CT colonography, also known as virtual colonoscopy, involves taking a series of X-rays to obtain detailed pictures of the colon and rectum. CT colonography is less intrusive than standard colonoscopy, but it still involves stool preparation and may miss tiny polyps or flat lesions.

In contrast, colonoscopy has various benefits, including the capacity to see the whole colon, remove polyps at the same time, and give a clear diagnosis. While colonoscopy involves intestinal preparation and anesthesia, the advantages of early identification and prevention of colorectal cancer exceed the procedure's momentary discomfort.

Long-Term Health Benefits And Implications

Colonoscopy has long-term health advantages beyond colorectal cancer prevention, including the diagnosis and treatment of other gastrointestinal diseases. A colonoscopy, which examines the colon for abnormalities, may help detect and treat illnesses including inflammatory bowel disease (IBD), diverticulosis, and colorectal polyps.

In addition to finding abnormalities, colonoscopy may be used to monitor persons with a history of colorectal cancer or precancerous polyps.

Regular surveillance colonoscopies enable physicians to watch for the return of cancer or new polyp development and act early if needed.

Furthermore, colonoscopy may give peace of mind to those who are at a higher risk of developing colorectal cancer owing to family history or genetics. By having frequent tests, these people may make proactive efforts to lower their risk of colorectal cancer and enhance their overall health.

While colonoscopy may seem intimidating to some, particularly owing to the needed intestinal preparation and anesthesia, the advantages greatly exceed the momentary pain involved with the procedure. Individuals who undergo regular colonoscopy screening may greatly lower their risk of colorectal cancer and other gastrointestinal disorders, resulting in improved long-term health and well-being.

CHAPTER 9

Special Considerations And FAQ

Colonoscopy For Those With Certain Medical Issues

Colonoscopy is a versatile diagnostic method that may identify a variety of problems in the colon and rectum. Individuals with certain medical issues, on the other hand, may need to take additional precautions before having the surgery.

Patients with heart issues, such as congestive heart failure or a history of heart attacks, may need additional monitoring during a colonoscopy owing to the use of sedatives and the possible pressure on the cardiovascular system. To guarantee a safe operation, these patients must have a full discussion of their medical history with their physician.

Similarly, people with respiratory disorders such as asthma or chronic obstructive pulmonary disease (COPD) should contact their doctor before undergoing a colonoscopy. Sedatives may impair breathing, therefore extra care may be required to handle any respiratory concerns during the surgery.

Individuals with diabetes must maintain their blood sugar levels before, during, and after a colonoscopy. Fasting before the treatment might impact blood glucose levels, therefore patients should follow their doctor's recommendations for medication modifications and food restrictions.

Patients with gastrointestinal disorders including inflammatory bowel disease (IBD) or diverticulitis may be more likely to have difficulties during a colonoscopy. In certain circumstances, these disorders might induce inflammation or constriction of the colon, complicating the surgery. Close collaboration between the gastroenterologist and the patient's primary care physician is required to provide a safe and successful colonoscopy.

Furthermore, those with a history of colorectal cancer or polyps may need more regular colonoscopies for monitoring reasons. These patients should collaborate with their healthcare practitioner to create a specific screening plan based on their medical history and risk factors.

In all circumstances, clear communication between the patient, gastroenterologist, and other healthcare personnel is critical to ensuring the safest and most successful colonoscopy possible.

Age Guidelines And Screening Frequency

The age at which people should begin regular colonoscopy screening is determined by a variety of variables, including their personal and family medical history.

In general, screening should begin at age 50 for average-risk adults who have no symptoms or predisposing circumstances.

Individuals with a family history of colorectal cancer or certain genetic diseases, such as familial adenomatous polyposis (FAP) or Lynch syndrome, may need earlier and more frequent screening. These people may undergo colonoscopies as early as age 40, or perhaps sooner, depending on their healthcare provider's precise recommendations.

The frequency of colonoscopy screening varies according to individual risk factors and prior screening results. A colonoscopy is normally suggested every ten years for those at moderate risk who have normal lab findings. However, people with a history of precancerous polyps or other abnormalities may need more regular tests, often every 3 to 5 years.

Individuals' chance of acquiring colorectal cancer rises with age, thus frequent screening is still crucial. When choosing the most suitable screening plan for older persons, healthcare experts will take into account aspects such as general health, life expectancy, and personal preferences.

Individuals should discuss their personal and family medical history with their healthcare practitioner to build a tailored screening strategy that suits their requirements and lowers their risk of colorectal cancer.

Addressing Frequent Worries And Anxieties

Colonoscopy is an effective technique for diagnosing colorectal cancer and other gastrointestinal disorders, but many individuals are concerned about the operation. Addressing these frequent concerns will help people feel more at ease and confident about their colonoscopy.

One typical issue is the pain caused by bowel preparation, which entails emptying the colon before the treatment. While stool prep may be difficult and uncomfortable, it is an important step in ensuring a successful colonoscopy because it allows for a clear view of the colon lining. Healthcare experts may give recommendations and guidance to make the bowel preparation process more comfortable, such as drinking lots of clear fluids and utilizing flavored laxatives.

Another source of worry is the use of sedation during colonoscopy, which increases the risk of problems or adverse effects. While sedatives are normally used to assist patients relax and reduce pain during the surgery, they may sometimes produce sleepiness, nausea, and other transitory side effects. Patients should address any concerns or medical issues with their healthcare professional before ensuring a safe and enjoyable experience.

Individuals scheduled for a colonoscopy often experience fear of the unknown. Giving patients extensive information about the surgery, including what to anticipate before, during, and after, may help reduce fear and uncertainty. Healthcare practitioners may assist patients to feel more at ease by answering questions, addressing worries, and providing comfort.

Finally, some people may be apprehensive about the findings of the colonoscopy, which might reveal colorectal cancer or other severe disorders. While it is reasonable to be concerned about the unknown, early identification with a colonoscopy may greatly improve results for colorectal cancer and other gastrointestinal diseases. To alleviate these worries, healthcare practitioners should highlight the need for screening as well as the possible advantages of early detection.

By addressing common worries and anxieties, healthcare practitioners may help patients feel more educated, prepared, and confident about having a colonoscopy.

Clearing Any Misunderstandings Regarding The Technique

Despite its usefulness in diagnosing colorectal cancer and other gastrointestinal disorders, colonoscopy is often misinterpreted or connected with myths. Clearing up these myths may help people make more informed choices about receiving the treatment.

One widespread myth is that colonoscopy is very painful and unpleasant. While it is reasonable to be nervous about any medical treatment, advances in anesthesia and technology have made colonoscopy far more manageable than in the past. Most patients feel little pain throughout the treatment, and they are often sedated to assist them relax and relieve any discomfort.

Another common myth is that colonoscopy is only essential for elderly persons or those who have colorectal cancer symptoms. In actuality, screening colonoscopy is suggested for average-risk adults beginning at age 50, even if symptoms are not present. Screening for colorectal cancer may help prevent it or discover it at an earlier, more curable stage.

There is also a misperception that other screening procedures, such as stool testing or virtual colonoscopy, are as effective as conventional colonoscopy. While these tests may be useful in specific instances, colonoscopy remains the gold standard for diagnosing and preventing colorectal cancer because it can view and remove precancerous polyps during the operation.

Some people may assume that a colonoscopy is unnecessary if they do not have a family history of colorectal cancer or other risk factors. However, many colorectal cancer instances occur in people who have no family history or obvious risk factors. Screening colonoscopy may help discover colorectal cancer or precancerous polyps in people who don't have clear risk factors, possibly saving lives via early diagnosis and treatment.

Healthcare practitioners may assist people make educated choices about their colorectal cancer screening options by dispelling myths and giving factual information about the advantages and necessity of colonoscopy.

CHAPTER 10

Moving Forward: Taking Control Of Your Health

The Need For Regular Screenings And Preventive Care

Regular screenings and preventative treatment are essential for preserving your entire health, particularly your colon and digestive system. Colonoscopy, in particular, is an important technique for identifying and preventing colorectal cancer, which is one of the major causes of cancer-related deaths globally. By having frequent tests, you may detect any possible problems early on, when they are most curable.

Colonoscopy is advised for those over the age of 50, but those with a family history of colorectal cancer or other risk factors should begin screening sooner. During a colonoscopy, a flexible tube (known as a colonoscope) is introduced into the rectum and directed into the colon. This enables the doctor to inspect the colon's lining for any abnormalities, such as polyps or tumors, that may signal the existence of cancer.

One of the primary advantages of colonoscopy is its capacity to both identify and prevent colorectal cancer. During the process, any worrisome growths (polyps) might be excised and submitted for biopsy. Polyps are often precancerous, which means they have the potential to develop into cancer over time. By removing them early, you may dramatically minimize your chances of having colorectal cancer in the future.

It is crucial to understand that a colonoscopy is not a one-time surgery. To successfully monitor your colon health, adhere to the established screening criteria and schedule frequent colonoscopies as directed by your physician. You may lower your chance of colorectal cancer by being proactive about your health and getting frequent checkups.

How To Maintain A Healthy Colon And Digestive System

Maintaining a healthy colon and digestive tract is important for general health and may lower your chance of getting colorectal cancer. While a colonoscopy is a crucial tool for early diagnosis and prevention, there are other things you can do in your everyday life to improve colon health.

First and foremost, a well-balanced diet high in fiber, fruits, and vegetables is essential for good digestion and regular bowel movements. Fiber bulks up stool and moves it more effectively through the colon, lowering the risk of constipation and other digestive disorders. Furthermore, keeping hydrated by consuming enough water might assist your digestive system in functioning properly.

Regular exercise is another key aspect in supporting colon health. Physical exercise stimulates the muscles in your digestive system, encouraging regular bowel movements and lowering the risk of constipation. Aim for at least 30 minutes of moderate activity most days of the week to maintain a healthy colon.

In addition to diet and exercise, you should avoid smoking and restrict your alcohol intake, since both may raise your chance of getting colorectal cancer. Smoking has been related to an increased risk of colon cancer, and excessive alcohol use may irritate the colon lining, increasing the chance of polyp development.

Finally, keeping up with prescribed tests, such as a colonoscopy, is critical for preserving colon health. Regular screenings enable early identification and intervention in colorectal cancer, which may greatly improve results. By embracing these lifestyle changes, you may improve your colon health and lower your risk of colorectal cancer.

Advocacy For Colon Cancer Awareness And Prevention

Advocating for colon cancer awareness and prevention is critical for increasing awareness of the value of frequent screenings and early diagnosis. Despite being largely preventable and treated when detected early, colorectal cancer is nevertheless one of the major causes of cancer-related deaths globally.

Sharing your personal screening and preventive experiences is one approach to raising awareness about colon cancer. By publicly discussing your own colonoscopy experiences and urging others to be screened, you may help decrease the stigma associated with colorectal cancer and empower others to take charge of their health.

Participating in community activities and fundraisers dedicated to colon cancer awareness may also help generate cash for research and support services for individuals afflicted by the illness.

Participating in advocacy initiatives allows you to have a meaningful influence on colon cancer prevention and help increase screening rates and results.

Educating people about the need for colon cancer screening and prevention is also essential for advocacy activities. By dispelling myths and misunderstandings regarding the advantages of colonoscopies and other screening procedures, you may urge people to prioritize their colon health.

Finally, advocating for colon cancer awareness and prevention is about enabling people to take charge of their health and make educated screening choices. By working together to increase awareness and support screening activities, we can help to reduce the impact of colorectal cancer on people and communities alike.

Resources For More Information And Support

Finding trustworthy information and support options is critical for anybody navigating colon cancer screening and prevention. Fortunately, there are several organizations and online tools available to guide and assist you every step of the road.

The American Cancer Society (ACS) is a good source of information about colon cancer screening. The ACS website provides detailed information on the many kinds of screening tests available, as well as recommendations for when to begin and how often to repeat screening depending on individual risk factors.

The Centers for Disease Control and Prevention (CDC) is another valuable resource, including educational resources and tools to encourage colon cancer awareness and prevention. The CDC website provides information on the signs and symptoms of colorectal cancer, as well as strategies for lowering your risk via lifestyle modifications and routine screenings.

For people looking for help from those who have gone through similar circumstances, internet networks and support groups may be beneficial. Websites such as CancerCare.org and the Colorectal Cancer Alliance provide online forums and support groups where people impacted by colon cancer may connect and share their tales and experiences.

In addition to internet resources, many healthcare practitioners give counseling and support to patients undergoing colon cancer screening and treatment. If you have any concerns regarding the screening procedure or need emotional support, please contact your healthcare physician.

Using these resources will provide you with the knowledge and support you need to confidently navigate colon cancer screening and prevention.

Conclusion

To summarize, a thorough knowledge of colonoscopy is critical for both patients and healthcare practitioners. This diagnostic method is critical for detecting, preventing, and treating a variety of colorectal illnesses, including colorectal cancer. This comprehensive guide to understanding colonoscopy highlights numerous crucial elements, highlighting its importance and advantages.

For starters, colonoscopy is a very efficient way to examine the colon and rectum. Its capacity to see the interior lining of the large intestine enables the diagnosis of anomalies such as polyps, cancers, inflammation, and other lesions. Early diagnosis of these abnormalities is critical since it allows for prompt intervention and may prevent benign growths from progressing to malignant ones.

Second, the preparatory phase is critical to the success of a colonoscopy. Adequate bowel preparation provides a clear view of the colon, increasing examination accuracy and lowering the probability of missing anomalies. Patients must carefully follow their healthcare provider's recommendations to ensure appropriate preparation.

Furthermore, advances in technology and procedures have considerably enhanced the safety and efficacy of colonoscopy. High-definition imaging, narrow-band imaging, and virtual colonoscopy are all examples of innovations that improve visualization and detection rates. Additionally, the availability of sedative alternatives improves patient comfort throughout the surgery, resulting in a favorable experience.

Furthermore, colonoscopy has a therapeutic purpose in addition to diagnostics. During the operation, polyps may be removed, biopsies obtained, and certain disorders, such as bleeding, addressed. This skill not only assists in the detection of colorectal illnesses, but it also has therapeutic applications, perhaps averting the emergence of more severe problems.

It is important to remember that, although colonoscopy is an effective tool in colorectal healthcare, it is not without limits and hazards. Complications such as bleeding, perforation, and sedation-related adverse responses are possible, although infrequent. However, the advantages of colonoscopy much exceed the dangers, particularly given its ability to identify and prevent colorectal cancer.

In conclusion, a thorough knowledge of colonoscopy enables people to make educated choices concerning their colorectal health. Patients and healthcare practitioners may optimize the advantages of this vital diagnostic and therapeutic technique by recognizing its relevance, following preparatory procedures, embracing technology improvements, and understanding its therapeutic potential. Colonoscopy is a cornerstone in the battle against colorectal illnesses thanks to ongoing research, education, and accessibility, saving lives and improving outcomes for countless people all over the globe.

THE END

www.ingramcontent.com/pod-product-compliance
Lightning Source LLC
Chambersburg PA
CBHW071839210526
45479CB00001B/200